Table of Contents

Asthma is an inflammatory disease of the airways to the lungs. It makes breathing difficult and can make some physical activities challenging or even impossible.

According to the Centers for Disease Control and Prevention (CDC), about 25 million AmericansTrusted Source have asthma. It's the most common chronic condition among American children: 1 child out of every 12Trusted Source has asthma.

To understand asthma, it's necessary to understand a little about what happens when you breathe. Normally, with every breath you take, air goes through your nose or mouth, down into your throat, and into your airways, eventually making it to your lungs.

There are lots of small air passages in your lungs that help deliver oxygen from the air into your bloodstream.

Asthma symptoms occur when the lining of your airways swells and the muscles around them tighten. Mucus then fills the airways, further reducing the amount of air that can pass through.

These conditions can then bring on an asthma "attack," which is the coughing and tightness in the chest that's typical of asthma.

BREAKFAST

1. Southwestern Casserole

Prep Time: 20 Minutes

Cook Time: 40 Minutes

Servings: 10

Ingredients

- 1 lb pork sausage
- 1 onion , finely chopped
- 1 red bell pepper large, chopped
- 15 oz black beans from the can, drained
- 4 oz green chili peppers , diced, from the can
- 1 ½ cups cheddar cheese , shredded
- ½ cup Mozzarella cheese , shredded
- 3 cups hash browns , frozen, raw, uncooked, completely defrosted
- 6 eggs
- ½ cup heavy cream
- 1 teaspoon chili powder

- 1 teaspoon ground cumin
- 1 tablespoon butter melted

Instructions

1. Preheat oven to 375 F.
2. In a large skillet, cook pork sausage together with finely chopped onions on medium heat until the sausage is cooked through and is no longer pink. Add chopped red bell pepper, black beans, and diced green chili peppers. Add half the spices (½ teaspoon of chili powder and ½ teaspoon of cumin) and mix everything up.
3. Add shredded cheddar cheese, shredded mozzarella cheese, and hash browns to the sausage mixture and mix them in.
4. In a small bowl, whisk eggs, heavy cream, and the remaining half of spices (½ teaspoon of chili powder and ½ teaspoon of cumin).
5. Use 2.8 L (3 quarts) rectangular baking dish - 11 inches long x 8.5 inches wide x 3 inches deep. Brush the bottom and the sides of the baking pan with 1 tablespoon of melted butter.

6. Add half the sausage mixture to the baking pan, and pour half of the egg mixture over the sausage mixture, carefully and evenly. Add the remaining half of the sausage mixture on top, and pour the remaining half of the egg mixture evenly over the sausage mixture.

7. Bake, uncovered for about 40-50 minutes. The casserole is ready when the eggs are set and no longer liquid in the center. Let the dish cool for about 30 minutes before slicing it.

Prep Time: 20 Minutes

Cook Time: 40 Minutes

Servings: 10

Ingredients

- 1 lb pork sausage , regular
- 1 onion , medium, finely chopped
- 1 ½ cups cheddar cheese shredded
- ½ cup mozzarella cheese shredded
- 2 cups broccoli florets , steamed or cooked and drained
- 4 cups hash browns , frozen, raw, uncooked, completely defrosted
- 6 eggs
- ½ cup heavy cream
- ¼ teaspoon black pepper
- 1 tablespoon butter , melted

Instructions

1. Preheat oven to 375 F.

2. In a large skillet, cook pork sausage together with finely chopped onions on medium heat until the sausage is cooked through and is no longer pink.

3. Add shredded cheddar cheese, shredded mozzarella cheese, and broccoli florets (steamed or cooked and drained) to the sausage mixture and mix them in. Add hash browns and mix them in.

4. In a small bowl, whisk eggs, heavy cream, and black pepper.

5. Use 2.8 L (3 quarts) rectangular baking dish - 11 inches long x 8.5 inches wide x 3 inches deep. Brush the bottom and the sides of the baking pan with 1 tablespoon of melted butter.

6. Add half the sausage mixture to the baking pan, and pour half of the egg mixture over the sausage mixture, carefully and evenly. Add the remaining half of the sausage mixture on top, and pour the remaining half of the egg mixture evenly over the sausage mixture.

7. Bake, uncovered for about 40-50 minutes. The casserole is ready when the eggs are set and no longer liquid in the center. Let the dish cool for about 30 minutes before slicing it.

Prep Time: 15 Minutes

Cook Time: 20 Minutes

Servings: 4

Ingredients

For flank steak:

- 4 cloves garlic
- 1 teaspoon salt
- ½ teaspoon cumin
- ¼ teaspoon pepper
- ¼ teaspoon parsley
- ¼ teaspoon sage
- ¼ teaspoon curry
- ¼ teaspoon paprika
- ¼ cup olive oil
- 1 lb flank steak

For eggs and assembly:

- 8 eggs
- 1 tablespoon olive oil
- 4 corn tortillas gluten free

- 2 cups guacamole (made out of 2 avocados, you can make your own from scratch, or use guacamole mix in a packet, etc.)
- ½ cup Cheddar cheese , shredded
- ½ cup Mozzarella cheese , shredded
- Salt and pepper

Instructions

How to cook flank steak:

1. Mince garlic with knife, set aside. Combine spices together in a small bowl.
2. Pat steak dry, then rub spices all over. Sprinkle minced garlic on both sides of the steak.
3. Heat large skillet on high heat. Once the skillet gets hot, add olive oil until it sizzles. Then add flank steak to the skillet and sear on high heat 3-4 minutes on each side for medium-rare, making sure you have garlic searing underneath steak or around steak.
4. Transfer steak to a cutting board and let it rest 10 minutes. Cut steak across the grain into relatively thin slices. Set aside.

Assemble breakfast flank steak and eggs:

1. Grease a large skillet (with Pam) and heat it on medium heat until hot. Crack each egg and pour onto the hot skillet. Depending on the size of the skillet you may fry from 2 to 4 eggs at the same time. Do not overcrowd the skillet. Cook until the whites of the eggs solidify and the yolks remain medium-rare. Using a wide flat spatula, transfer eggs onto the plate.

2. In a large skillet fry tortillas in 1 tablespoon olive oil on both sides, until each tortilla puffs up. Place 4 tortilla on 4 serving plates.

3. Divide guacamole into 4 equal parts and put on top of each tortilla.

4. Top guacamole with slices of flank steak. Then top steak slices on each plate with 2 tablespoons of shredded cheddar and 2 tablespoons of shredded mozzarella. Finally, top each portion with 2 eggs cooked over easy. Sprinkle salt and pepper on top of eggs for taste and presentation.

Prep Time: 15 Minutes

Cook Time: 15 Minutes

Servings: 4

Ingredients

- 2 tablespoons olive oil
- 1 pound asparagus
- 8 eggs
- ¼ cup Half and Half
- 8 ounces goat cheese
- 8 slices bread whole grain or whole wheat

Instructions

1. Roasted Asparagus
2. Pre-heat the oven to 400 Fahrenheit. Trim ends of the asparagus. In a large bowl, toss asparagus with olive oil. Line a baking sheet with foil and place the asparagus on a baking sheet in a single layer. Season with salt and pepper. Roast the asparagus for 15 minutes: when it's done, it should be soft but crunchy.

Alternatively, if you don't want to turn on the oven, you can roast asparagus in a large frying pan on stove top for 10 minutes.

3. Scrambled Eggs

4. Whisk eggs with half and half until nice and fluffy. Spray a large skillet with non-stick spray, heat on medium heat, add whisked eggs and cook, on medium heat, stirring all the time using a heat-proof spatula or a wooden spoon. Cook until eggs are cooked through but are still soft and fluffy, not hardened. Sprinkle goat cheese on top of the scrambled eggs. Cover the skillet with the lid and remove from heat.

5. Assemble Sandwiches

6. Toast bread slices. Place 4 toasted bread slices on a working surface. Add ¼ of scrambled eggs (with melted goat cheese on top) on top of each bread slice. Top scrambled eggs with roasted asparagus (whole, or sliced in halves or quarters). Top with the remaining slice of bread or serve them as open sandwiches!

Prep Time: 20 Minutes

Cook Time: 10 Minutes

Servings: 4

Ingredients

Crepes:

- homemade crepes
- gluten free crepes
- 6 eggs or more
- Southwestern salsa
- 1 cup black beans , from the can, rinsed and drained
- ½ cup sweet yellow corn , from the can, rinsed and drained
- 1 cup tomato , chopped
- 1 red bell pepper , chopped in small cubes
- 1 green bell pepper , chopped in small cubes
- ¼ cup cilantro , chopped finely
- 2 tablespoons freshly squeezed lime juice
- Salt and pepper to taste

Instructions

Crepes:

1. Make classic French-style crepes according to this recipe. Or, make gluten free crepes according to this recipe.

Southwestern salsa:

2. In a large bowl, mix black beans, yellow corn, chopped tomato, chopped bell peppers. Add lime juice and salt and pepper to taste, mix well. Set aside to let the juices combine together.

Eggs:

1. Grease a large skillet with cooking spray, and heat the skillet on medium heat until hot. Crack each egg and pour onto the hot skillet. Depending on the size of the skillet you may fry from 2 to 4 eggs at the same time. Do not overcrowd the skillet. Cook until the whites of the eggs solidify and the yolks remain medium-rare. Using a wide flat spatula, transfer eggs onto the plate. Note Make the eggs only right before you are ready to assemble the dish (that is, after you made crepes and the Southwestern salsa), so that they don't get cold.

Assemble breakfast crepes

2. Place a crepe on a plate. Put some Southwestern salsa (you can warm it up or serve it at room temperature) on one half of the crepe. Top with a fried egg. Fold 3 sides of the crepe inwards to form a half-closed, half-open pocket as on the.

Prep Time: 30 Minutes

Cook Time: 1hr 10 Minutes

Servings: 6

Ingredients

For tart crust (6 mini tart shells, 3 inch diameter each):

- 1 ½ cups flour
- ¼ teaspoon salt
- 9 tablespoons unsalted butter cold
- 1 egg yolks
- 1 tablespoon ice water

For filling:

- 2 eggs
- ½ cup heavy cream
- ¼ cup milk
- ⅓ cup Gouda cheese shredded
- ⅛ teaspoon salt
- 1 tablespoon olive oil

- 5 oz spinach

- 20 grape tomatoes , yellow and red

- salt to taste

Instructions

Preparing tart shells (6 tart shells, 3 inch diameter each):

1. Prepare savory tart crust using the recipe and the method described in my recipe here. The only thing different here will be the size of tart pan: instead of using one large tart pan, use 6 smaller individual tartlet pans (3 inch diameter each). Bake empty smaller tart shells for about 20 minutes. You don't need to bake them to brown or golden color, because you will continue baking them once you put the filling in.

To make the filling:

2. Preheat oven to 350 F.
3. In a small skillet on stove top, cook spinach in olive oil for 10-15 minutes on medium heat until wilted. Salt to taste. Let it cool.
4. In a small bowl, whisk together eggs, heavy cream, milk. Then, add cheese and salt and mix well.

5. Divide spinach into 6 equal parts and place it in each of the baked 3″ tartlet shells, that you pre-baked in step 1. Divide the egg mixture into 6 equal parts and pour it over spinach into each of 6 tart shells.

6. Cut each grape tomato in half. Arrange tomato halves on top of each little tart, cut side down. As you see from the photo, the tart filling does not come all the way to the top of the tart shell edges, which is how it should be because the egg mixture will rise during baking.

7. Bake these egg tartlets for 20-30 minutes, until tart shell is golden brown and the filling top turns yellow-brownish and starts to rise, or when the tooth pick inserted in the middle of the tart comes out clean.

8. Remove from oven and let the tartlets cool for 10 minutes on wire rack before serving.

Prep Time: 30 Minutes

Cook Time: 1hr 25 Minutes

Servings: 6

Ingredients

For 6 tartlets (mini tart shells):

- 1 ½ cups flour
- ¼ teaspoon salt
- 9 tablespoons unsalted butter cold
- 1 egg yolks
- 1 tablespoon ice water

For filling:

- 1 egg
- ½ cup heavy cream
- ¼ cup milk
- ⅓ cup Gouda cheese , shredded
- 4 slices bacon , already cooked and chopped
- ⅛ teaspoon salt
- 1 tablespoon olive oil

- 5 oz spinach
- 6 eggs
- salt to taste

Instructions

1. How to make tartlets (6 mini tart shells, 3 inch diameter each):
2. Prepare savory tart crust using the recipe and the method described in my recipe here. The only thing different here will be the size of tart pan: instead of using one large tart pan, use 6 smaller individual tartlet pans (3 inch diameter each). Bake empty smaller tart shells for about 20 minutes. You don't need to bake them to brown or golden color, because you will continue baking them once you put the filling in.

How to make breakfast filling:

1. Preheat oven to 350 F.
2. Cook spinach in olive oil for 10-15 minutes on medium heat until wilted. Salt to taste. Let it cool. Make sure to drain any liquid resulting from cooking spinach.

3. In a small bowl, whisk together 1 egg, heavy cream, milk. Add shredded cheese, bacon (cooked and chopped finely), and salt and mix well.

4. Divide spinach into 6 equal parts and place each spinach portion in each of the 3″ tartlet shells, that you pre-baked in step 1. Divide the egg mixture from step 3 into 6 equal parts and pour each portion over spinach into each of 6 tartlets.

5. Crack an egg over each mini tart shell (6 eggs for 6 tartlets in this recipe). Season with salt, pepper.

6. Bake these tartlets for 20-30 minutes, until tart shell is golden brown and eggs are almost set.

7. Remove from oven and let it cool for 10 minutes on wire rack before serving.

Prep Time: 1hrs 10 Minutes

Cook Time: 1hr 05 Minutes

Servings: 10

Ingredients

For tart crust:

- 1 ½ cups flour
- ¼ teaspoon salt
- 9 tablespoons unsalted butter cold
- 1 egg yolks
- 1 tablespoon ice water

Ingredients for tart filling:

- ½ cup leek chopped
- 1 tablespoon olive oil
- 3 sprigs thyme fresh
- 2 eggs
- ½ cup heavy cream
- ¼ cup milk
- ⅓ cup Gruyere cheese shredded

- ⅛ teaspoon salt
- 20 grape tomatoes yellow and red

Instructions

How to make savory tart shell:

1. Prepare and bake savory tart dough according to my recipe. Cool completely.
2. Savory tart filling:
3. Preheat oven to 350 F.
4. In a skillet on a stove top, cook chopped leeks in olive oil for 10 minutes until softened. Add finely chopped thyme to leeks. Let it cool.
5. In a small bowl, whisk together eggs, heavy cream, milk. Then, add cheese, leeks mixture, and salt and mix well.
6. Pour the mixture into the cooled tart shell, distributing leeks evenly. As you see on the photo below, the mixture does not come to the top of the tart shell edges, which is normal. Once it's cooked, the egg mixture will actually rise.
7. Cut grape tomatoes in half. Arrange them on top of the tart, cut side down.

8. Bake tart for 50 minutes, until tart shell is golden brown and the filling top turns yellow-brownish and starts to rise, or when the tooth pick inserted in the middle of the tart comes out clean. Remove from oven and let it cool for 10 minutes on wire rack before serving.

Prep Time: 15 Minutes

Cook Time: 55 Minutes

Servings: 6

Ingredients

Peach and blueberry filling

- 4 peaches cored, unpeeled, sliced into wedges
- 12 oz blueberries
- 4 tablespoons salted butter melted
- ½ fresh lemon squeezed
- ⅓ cup brown sugar
- 1 teaspoon vanilla extract
- 1 tablespoon cornstarch

Crisp topping

- ¼ cup all-purpose flour
- ¾ cup oats old-fashioned rolled or regular or quick
- ½ cup almonds sliced and toasted
- ½ cup brown sugar
- 5 tablespoons salted butter softened not melted

Instructions

1. Preheat the oven
2. Preheat the oven to 375 F.
3. Use a 10 x 7 inch high-sided, rectangular baking dish. Or use a 10-inch high-sided cast-iron skillet or 9-inch or 10-inch high-sided round baking dish.

Make a crisp filling

1. In a large bowl, combine melted butter, sliced peaches, blueberries, freshly squeezed lemon juice, brown sugar, vanilla extract, and cornstarch. Mix really well with the spoon, being careful not to break the fruit. Reserve some of the sliced peaches and blueberries for later use.
2. Transfer the fruit mixture to a butter-greased baking dish.

Make a topping

1. In a medium mixing bowl, combine flour, oats, and toasted sliced almonds. Add the softened (not melted) butter and use a fork to work the butter into the dry ingredients until everything is moist and clumps together.

2. Sprinkle the topping over the fruit mixture in a baking
    dish. Scatter the reserved sliced peaches and
    blueberries around the edges of the crisp.

Bake

1. Transfer the peach and blueberry crisp to the oven
    and bake, uncovered, for 40 or 45 minutes or until the
    top is golden and the fruit is bubbling.
2. Remove from the oven and let cool slightly.

Prep Time: 20 Minutes

Cook Time: 1hrs 15 Minutes

Servings: 12

Ingredients

- 1 ½ cups all-purpose flour
- 1 teaspoon baking powder
- ½ teaspoon baking soda
- 2 oz butter softened (4 tablespoons)
- 1 cup sugar
- 2 eggs
- ½ teaspoon vanilla
- ½ cup sour cream
- 4 peaches medium, sliced into wedges
- 6 oz blueberries

Instructions

1. I used 10-inch round high-sided cast-iron skillet. You can also use a regular 8-inch or 9-inch round cake pan or a 9x3-inch springform pan.

2. Preheat oven to 350°F with rack in middle. Grease the sides and the bottom of the cast-iron pan with butter.

3. Sift flour, baking powder, baking soda, together into a medium bowl.

4. In a separate bowl, beat 2 oz of softened butter, sugar, and 2 eggs until very light in color and fluffy, 2-3 minutes on high speed.

5. Add vanilla and Greek yogurt and continue beating until very creamy and light in color, for about 1 more minute.

6. Keeping the mixer speed low, mix in the flour mix until combined. Do not overmix.

7. Transfer the cake batter to the cast-iron skillet. Top with sliced peaches, and scatter blueberries evenly on top in the spaces between the peach slices.

8. Bake uncovered until the cake turns golden, and the tester comes out clean in the center, about 45 minutes to 1 hour, depending on your oven. Midway through baking, I like to put some extra peach slices and extra blueberries on top of the cake for presentation purposes, and return the cake to baking.

9. When the cake is done baking, remove it from the oven and let it cool in a cast-iron skillet.

11. Cilantro-Lime Chicken Bowls with Peach Salsa

Prep Time: 15 Minutes

Cook Time: 15 Minutes

Servings: 4

Ingredients

Peach Salsa:

- 3 yellow peaches medium size, pitted and diced
- 1 sweet red bell pepper diced
- ¼ cup red onion diced
- 3 green onions finely chopped
- ½ bunch cilantro chopped
- 2 tablespoons freshly squeezed lime juice or more
- ¼ teaspoon chili powder or more
- ¼ teaspoon salt or more to taste

Cilantro-Lime Honey Chicken

- 1 lb chicken breasts skinless, boneless, sliced
- ½ teaspoon smoked paprika
- 1 teaspoon chili powder

- ¼ teaspoon salt to taste

- freshly ground black pepper

- 2 tablespoons olive oil

- 2 tablespoons freshly squeezed lime juice (juice from ½ lime)

- 2 tablespoons honey

- 1 tablespoon butter

Rice:

- 2 cups cooked rice I used Jasmine rice

- Garnish

- Fresh cilantro chopped

- 1 lime sliced

Instructions

How to make peach salsa

1. About peaches. Wash them thoroughly to get rid of any debris. There is no need to peel the peaches. Chop them carefully to keep the skin on.

2. In a large mixing bowl combine all fruit salsa ingredients. Toss to combine. Taste and season with salt and pepper, if needed. Add more lime juice and chili powder, if you like.

3. How to make cilantro-lime chicken

4. Generously season the sliced chicken breasts with salt, pepper, smoked paprika, and chili powder.

5. Heat 2 tablespoons of olive oil in a large skillet over medium-high heat. When the oil is hot, add sliced skinless boneless chicken breasts. Cook, undisturbed, for about 4 minutes, to let chicken sear.

6. Flip the chicken strips over and cook for 2 more minutes. Lower the heat to low, add freshly squeezed lime juice and honey. Cook for another 2 minutes or more, frequently stirring, until the chicken is cooked through.

7. Remove from heat. Add 2 tablespoons of butter to the skillet and stir, off heat, to coat the chicken. Stir in the chopped fresh parsley.

Assembly

1. Add cooked jasmine rice to the bowls. Spoon the peach salsa and the cilantro-lime honey chicken over the rice. Top with chopped fresh cilantro and fresh lime slices.

Prep Time: 15 Minutes

Cook Time: 15 Minutes

Servings: 4

Ingredients

Simple sweet chili sauce:

- 2 tablespoons rice vinegar
- 2 tablespoons soy sauce
- ⅓ cup fig spread or more, for thickening the glaze (I prefer to use Divina brand)
- red pepper flakes to taste

Salmon:

- 24 oz salmon fillets (4 salmon fillets)
- 2 tablespoons olive oil
- 2 cloves garlic minced
- salt and pepper

Mango salsa:

- 2 mangos mangos ripe, peeled, pitted, and diced
- 1 sweet red bell pepper small, diced

- ½ bunch fresh cilantro chopped
- 2 tablespoons freshly squeezed lime juice
- ¼ teaspoon chili powder or more
- salt and pepper to taste

Rice:

- 2 cups cooked rice I used Jasmine rice
- Garnish
- 1 lime sliced
- fresh cilantro chopped

Instructions

2. Preheat the oven to 425 F.
3. Make the sweet chili sauce
4. Combine all the ingredients for the sauce in a small bowl and mix well.

Cook the salmon:

1. Use whole salmon fillets or slice each into 3 chunks. Season the salmon with olive oil, minced garlic, salt, and pepper. Spread in a single layer in a baking dish skin-side down.

2. Roast for about 10 or 12 minutes in the preheated oven at 425 F or until the salmon is almost cooked through.

3. Remove from the oven. At this point, if you don't like the salmon skin, remove it by sliding a spatula carefully under each salmon fillet or chunk to separate the fillet from the skin. Discard the skin. Or leave the skin on!

4. Coat the salmon with the sticky sweet chili glaze (reserving about ⅓ of the sauce for later) and return briefly to the oven to continue cooking (a couple of minutes) until the salmon is cooked through.

5. While the salmon is roasted in the oven, proceed with the rest of the recipe and prepare the mango salsa and the bowls.

Mango salsa:

1. About mangos. Wash them thoroughly to get rid of any debris. Use ripe mangos. Always peel the mangos. Pit the mangos and dice them into cubes.

2. In a medium mixing bowl combine diced mangos, diced red bell pepper, chopped fresh cilantro, freshly squeezed lime juice, and chili powder. Toss to combine.

Assembly:

1. Add cooked jasmine rice to the bowls. Top with glazed salmon on one side and mango salsa on the other side. Glaze the salmon with the reserved ⅓ of sweet chili sauce. Top with chopped fresh cilantro and fresh lime slices.

Prep Time: 20 Minutes

Cook Time: 25 Minutes

Servings: 4

Ingredients

Pasta:

- 8 oz pasta such as fettuccine, pappardelle, egg pasta, or rice noodles
- 1 tablespoon extra virgin olive oil
- salt to taste
- Salmon:
- 24 oz salmon fillets (4 salmon fillets)
- 4 cloves garlic minced
- salt to taste
- 2 tablespoons butter

Asian glaze:

- 2 tablespoons fish sauce (I prefer to use anchovy-based fish sauce)
- 3 tablespoons low-sodium soy sauce or tamari sauce
- 2 tablespoons rice vinegar

- ⅓ cup fig spread or more, for thickening the glaze (I prefer to use Divina brand)
- red pepper flakes to taste

Mango peach salsa:

- 2 mangos ripe, peeled, pitted, and diced
- 2 peaches cored and diced
- 1 sweet red bell pepper small, diced
- ½ bunch fresh cilantro chopped
- 2 tablespoons freshly squeezed lime juice
- ¼ teaspoon chili powder or more
- salt and pepper to taste

Instructions

Cook pasta

1. Bring a pot of water to boil. Add pasta and cook according to package instructions.
2. When pasta is done, drain. Add olive oil to the pasta and a pinch of salt, and toss together.
3. Proceed with the rest of the recipe while the pasta is cooking.

Cook the salmon

1. Preheat the oven to 375 F.

2. Grease the bottom of the baking dish with butter. Add salmon fillets skin side down.

3. Sprinkle the salmon with salt and minced garlic on top and around. Add thin slices of butter on top of each salmon fillet.

4. Bake for about 12 or 15 minutes. Remove from the oven.

5. if you would like to pan-sear the salmon on the stovetop instead, see instructions in the Recipe How to make the Asian glaze

6. While the salmon is baking and the pasta is cooking, prepare the glaze.

7. In a medium, high-sided bowl, combine the Asian glaze ingredients. Mix everything well. Sprinkle with red pepper flakes to taste.

8. Spread the glaze over each salmon fillet (after the salmon has been baked for 12 or 15 minutes). Note: Reserve half or ⅓ of the glaze for pouring over pasta.

9. Return the salmon to the oven for about 2 or 5 minutes or until the salmon is cooked to your likeness.

10. Salmon is done when it flakes easily with the fork and the internal temperature measures 145 degrees F on an instant-read thermometer.

11. Make mango peach salsa

12. Prepare the mango peach salsa while the salmon is baking.

13. Note about mangos. Wash them thoroughly to get rid of any debris. Use ripe mangos. Always peel the mangos. Pit the mangos and dice them into cubes.

14. In a large mixing bowl combine diced mangos, diced peaches, diced red bell pepper, and chopped fresh cilantro. Toss to combine.

15. Add freshly squeezed lime juice and chili powder. Toss to combine. Taste and season with salt and pepper, if needed. Add more lime juice and chili powder, if you like.

Assembly

1. In each serving bowl, combine cooked pasta together with cooked salmon.

2. Spoon mango peach salsa next to or over the baked salmon.

3. Spoon the reserved Asian glaze over the pasta and salmon.

4. Top with chopped fresh cilantro.

Prep Time: 20 Minutes

Cook Time: 10 Minutes

Servings: 6

Ingredients

Corn pasta salad:

- 8 oz orecchiette pasta or other short pasta
- 1 cup corn kernels cooked
- 1 red bell pepper diced
- 4 slices bacon cooked and sliced
- fresh cilantro chopped
- salt and pepper to taste

Salad dressing

- ⅓ cup basil pesto store-bought or homemade
- 3 tablespoons Greek yogurt
- 2 tablespoons mayonnaise
- 2 tablespoons lime juice freshly squeezed

Instructions

Cook pasta:

1. Bring a pot of water to boil. Add pasta and cook according to package instructions. Drain.
2. While the pasta is cooking, proceed with the rest of the recipe.
3. Make salad dressing
4. In a mason jar, whisk together basil pesto with Greek yogurt, mayonnaise, and freshly squeezed lime juice.
5. If your dressing is too thick, you can thin it out by adding more Greek yogurt, small amounts of water, or extra lime juice (or lemon juice). Or, combination of what I just listed.

Assembly

1. In a large bowl, combine cooked and drained pasta, cooked corn kernels, diced bell pepper, and chopped cooked bacon. Mix to combine.
2. Distribute into individual salad bowls. Top with the salad dressing. Sprinkle the chopped fresh cilantro on top.

Prep Time: 15 Minutes

Cook Time: 15 Minutes

Servings: 4

Ingredients

- 8 oz fusilli spiral pasta or use rotini, farfalle (bow-tie), penne, or rigatoni
- 3 ears corn on the cob or use canned corn
- Other salad ingredients
- 1 red bell pepper diced
- ½ cup black beans from the can, drained and rinsed (½ can - 83 grams)
- ½ cup Cotija cheese grated
- ½ bunch cilantro chopped

Salad dressing:

- ¼ cup mayonnaise
- ½ cup Greek yogurt
- 1 small lime freshly squeezed or more to taste
- 2 tablespoons sriracha sauce
- 1 teaspoon chili powder or more

- cayenne pepper to taste (use it sparingly, it adds heat fast)
- salt and pepper to taste

Garnish

- 4 green onions chopped
- chili powder to taste

Instructions

Cook pasta:

1. Bring a large pot of water to boil. Add pasta and cook pasta al dente according to the package instructions. While the pasta is cooking, proceed with the rest of the recipe.
2. When the pasta is done, drain.
3. Cook corn
4. You can either grill the corn on the cob or boil it in the pot of water on the stovetop. Or, simply use canned corn kernels.
5. How to grill it. Remove the husks and the silks from corn on the cob. Preheat your outdoor grill to medium-high heat. Brush corn with olive oil, salt, and pepper all over. Grill until lightly charred for about 10

or 15 minutes. Rotate the corn frequently while grilling. Let it cool. Once cooled off, slice the corn kernels off the cob with the knife.

6. How to boil it. Bring a large pot of water to boil. Remove the husks and the silks from corn on the cob. Boil the corn for about 5 or 10 minutes until cooked. Remove it from the pot and let it cool. Once cooled off, slice the corn kernels off the cob with the knife.

Make the salad dressing

1. Combine all salad dressing ingredients in a mason jar. Whisk well with a fork.
2. use cayenne pepper to taste and use sparingly as it adds heat fast. Skip it if you don't like things too spicy.

Assembly

1. In a large mixing bowl, combine cooked and drained pasta, cooked corn kernels, diced bell pepper, drained black beans, grated Cotija cheese, and chopped fresh cilantro. Mix.
2. Add salad dressing and mix to combine. Season with salt and pepper.
3. When serving, top with chopped green onions and sprinkle with chili powder. You can also sprinkle the salad with extra cheese if you like.

Prep Time: 20 Minutes

Cook Time: 10 Minutes

Servings: 4

Ingredients

Creamy Cilantro-Lime Salad Dressing

- ½ cup Greek yogurt or sour cream
- ¼ cup mayonnaise
- 2 tablespoons lime juice freshly squeezed
- 1 tablespoon Dijon mustard
- ¼ cup fresh cilantro finely chopped
- 1 tablespoon olive oil
- 1 clove garlic minced

Salad Ingredients

- 2 ears sweet corn husks and silks removed (corn on the cob)
- 10 oz cherry tomatoes halved
- 1 avocado diced

* 3 slices bacon cooked, chopped (optional)
* ⅓ cup feta cheese crumbled
* ⅓ cup fresh cilantro finely chopped

Instructions

1. In a mason jar, combine all salad dressing ingredients and whisk together well.
2. Bring a pot of water to boil. Cook corn for about 5 minutes. Remove from heat, and drain. Let it cool. Cut corn kernels off the cob with the knife.
3. In a large bowl, combine corn kernels, halved cherry tomatoes, diced avocado, chopped cooked bacon (optional), crumbled feta cheese, half of chopped cilantro. Toss lightly to combine.
4. Distribute the salad into individual salad bowls. Top with the creamy cilantro-lime salad dressing. Sprinkle the remaining chopped fresh cilantro on top.

Prep Time: 30 Minutes

Cook Time: 25 Minutes

Servings: 6

Ingredients

- 1 tablespoon olive oil
- 1 pound ground beef
- 1 lb butternut squash peeled and chopped into ¾ inch cubes (¼ of whole squash or 2 cups chopped squash)
- 1 green bell pepper chopped
- 4 garlic cloves minced
- 15 oz red kidney beans from the can, rinsed
- oz corn from the can, rinsed
- 28 oz tomatoes from the can (I used peeled tomatoes Cento San Marzano brand)
- 2 cups water
- 1 tablespoon chili powder
- 1 tablespoon cumin
- 1 teaspoon sugar
- ½ teaspoon salt at least

For garnish:

- ¼ cup cheddar cheese shredded
- 4 green onions chopped
- ¼ cup Greek yogurt

Instructions

1. Heat olive oil in a large skillet. Add ground beef and cook until no longer pink. Drain the ground beef of any fat.
2. To the same pan, add cubed butternut squash, chopped green bell pepper, minced garlic, kidney beans, corn, and canned tomatoes.
3. Use a spoon to break all tomatoes into small bites.
4. Add 2 cups of water.
5. Season with 1 tablespoon chili powder, 1 tablespoon cumin, 1 teaspoon of sugar, and salt to taste (at least ½ teaspoon of salt).
6. Mix everything well, and bring to boil. Reduce to simmer. Cook on low simmer for about 20-25 minutes until squash is tender. Remove from heat.
7. Add extra chili powder, if you want more heat. Season with more salt, if necessary.

8. Serve topped with shredded cheddar cheese, chopped green onions, and a dollop of Greek yogurt.

Prep Time: 10 Minutes

Cook Time: 25 Minutes

Servings: 4

Ingredients

- 4 chicken breasts
- ½ pound asparagus chopped into thirds (2-inch slices)
- 6 strips bacon cooked, chopped
- ½ cup Ranch dressing
- 1 cup Cheddar cheese shredded

Instructions

1. Preheat oven to 375 F.
2. Add chicken breasts to the casserole dish.
3. Add chopped asparagus all around and on top of the chicken.
4. Add chopped cooked bacon around and on top of the chicken.
5. Spread Ranch dressing over the chicken breasts.

6. Top with shredded Cheddar cheese.

7. Bake, uncovered, for 25-30 minutes, until the chicken is cooked through. Broil for the last 4 minutes if desired.

Prep Time: 15 Minutes

Cook Time: 30 Minutes

Servings: 4

Ingredients

Cajun Seasoning:

- 1 teaspoon paprika
- ¼ teaspoon cayenne pepper
- ¼ teaspoon oregano
- ¼ teaspoon thyme
- ¼ teaspoon salt

Chicken:

- 2 bell peppers , small, thinly sliced (or use mini sweet peppers)
- 4 chicken breasts , small
- 4 cloves garlic , minced
- 6 oz cream cheese , cold, refrigerated, and sliced into 8 slices
- ½ cup cheddar cheese , shredded

Instructions

1. How to make Cajun chicken seasoning
2. Combine all seasoning ingredients in a small bowl. Mix to combine.

Cajun chicken

1. Preheat oven to 375 F.
2. Place thinly sliced bell peppers on the bottom of the casserole dish.
3. Place chicken breasts on top (so that the peppers will cook underneath the chicken).
4. Generously sprinkle Cajun seasoning all over the chicken breasts. You don't have to use all the seasoning.   Top with minced garlic.
5. Top each chicken breast with 2 slices of cream cheese.
6. Top with shredded cheddar cheese.
7. Bake the chicken uncovered at 375 F in the preheated oven for 20-30 minutes until the chicken is cooked through.
8. Broil for 2 minutes, if desired.
9. To serve, scoop the bell peppers from underneath the chicken. Place them evenly around the chicken and on top.

Prep Time: 20 Minutes

Cook Time: 20 Minutes

Servings: 5

Ingredients

- 2 tablespoons olive oil
- 1 lb Italian sausages , casings removed, sliced
- 1 small onion , very finely chopped
- 4 garlic cloves , finely minced
- 1 tablespoon Cajun seasoning
- 1 bell pepper , very finely chopped
- 4 tomatoes , chopped, or 15 cherry tomatoes, each sliced in half
- 8 ounces mushrooms , finely sliced
- ¾ cup red wine
- 10 oz penne pasta (for gluten-free, use gluten-free brown rice penne)
- ½ cup Parmesan cheese , shredded

Instructions

1. Remove casings from the sausage and slice the sausage into small pieces.

2. In a large skillet, heat 1 tablespoon of olive oil and add sausage. Cook, occasionally stirring, until it's cooked through, drain the fat. Add another tablespoon of olive oil into the skillet with sausage, add chopped onion and garlic, half of the Cajun seasoning - cook, constantly stirring, on high heat until onion softens.

3. Add chopped bell peppers, tomatoes, mushrooms, and the remaining half of Cajun seasoning to the skillet with sausage. Cook for about 2 minutes, constantly stirring, on medium-high heat to sear the vegetables nicely on stove-top.

4. Add wine to the skillet, bring to boil, reduce to simmer and simmer, covered, occasionally stirring, for about 5-7 minutes. The liquid should reduce somewhat but not completely. Remove from heat. Salt to taste. Add more Cajun seasoning, if necessary.

5. Cook pasta al dente according to package instructions. Drain and immediately add to the skillet with the sauce. Mix everything well, cover, and heat the pasta on low heat for 1-2 minutes.

6. To serve, sprinkle with grated Parmesan cheese and
   black pepper.

21. Creamy Broccoli and Cauliflower Salad

Prep Time: 20 Minutes

Cook Time: 10 Minutes

Servings: 8

Ingredients

Broccoli and Cauliflower Salad:

- 3 cups broccoli florets finely chopped into small pieces
- 3 cups cauliflower florets finely chopped into small pieces
- 1 cup carrots finely sliced
- ½ cup red onion diced
- 10 slices bacon cooked, drained of fat, and chopped
- 1 cup sharp cheddar cheese shredded
- 1 cup dried cranberries

Salad Dressing:

- ½ cup mayonnaise
- ½ cup sour cream or kefir or Greek yogurt
- 2 tablespoons lemon juice

- ¼ cup honey softened or warmed up
- ¼ teaspoon salt

Instructions

Broccoli and Cauliflower Salad:

1. In a large bowl, combine together all salad ingredients.

Salad Dressing:

2. In a small bowl, stir together mayonnaise, sour cream (or kefir or Greek yogurt), lemon juice, honey, and salt. Note that honey should be soft and runny, warm it up if needed so that it mixes easily. Whisk the ingredients until well combined and smooth. Add salt if needed.
3. Gradually add the salad dressing to the large bowl with the salad ingredients, and stir everything together.

Prep Time: 30 Minutes

Cook Time: 10 Minutes

Servings: 4

Ingredients

Greek Salad Dressing:

- ¼ cup olive oil
- ¼ cup balsamic vinegar or 2 tablespoons each balsamic and red wine vinegar
- ¼ teaspoon ground black pepper or more, to taste
- ¼ teaspoon salt or more, to taste
- ½ teaspoon white sugar
- 2 tablespoons Greek yogurt optional

Salad Ingredients:

- 2 cucumbers , sliced thinly
- 3 avocados , peeled, cored, and cubed
- 7 oz cheese tortellini , uncooked
- 1 cup feta cheese , crumbled

Instructions

How to make Greek salad dressing:

1. In a medium bowl, whisk together olive oil, vinegar(s), black pepper, salt, and sugar. Add a tablespoon of Greek yogurt for a little creaminess

How to make salad:

2. Cook tortellini according to package instructions, drain and let them cool.
3. In a large mixing bowl, combine cooked tortellini, sliced cucumber, cubed avocados, feta cheese.
4. Add just enough of the dressing to the salad to coat and toss (start with adding half the amount of dressing). Don't add all the salad dressing at once.
5. Cover and chill for a couple of hours or refrigerate overnight. Also chill (or refrigerate) the remaining dressing.
6. Before serving, let the salad (and the remaining dressing) sit at room temperature for some time because olive oil in the dressing would've have solidified in the refrigerator - let it liquify. Add more of the reserved dressing to the salad, if necessary.

Prep Time: 20 Minutes

Cook Time: 30 Minutes

Servings: 4

Ingredients

- 1 tablespoon olive oil
- 0.4 lb smoked sausage , sliced (I used Gyulai Smoked Sausage)
- ¼ cup sun-dried tomatoes , without oil, finely chopped
- 4 garlic cloves , minced
- 1 ½ cups half and half
- 1 cup mozzarella cheese , shredded
- 8 oz penne pasta
- ¼ teaspoon red pepper flakes
- salt to taste (optional)

Instructions

1. Heat olive oil in a large skillet on medium-high heat. Add sliced sausage, cook for 4 minutes, about 2

minutes on each side. Sausage will release its own juice. Remove sausage from the skillet.

2. To the same skillet, add chopped sun-dried tomatoes and minced garlic. Cook for about 1 minute, constantly stirring.

3. Add half and half. Bring to boil. Add cheese, reduce heat, and keep stirring until the cheese melts. Bring heat to medium, if needed, to melt the cheese, then reduce to simmer.

4. Cook pasta, drain.

5. Add cooked and drained pasta and sausage back to the skillet with the sauce. Stir. Add pepper flakes.

6. Note: I did not have to add salt, as the smoked sausage is already salty and provides enough saltiness. Add salt to taste, if needed.

Prep Time: 20 Minutes

Cook Time: 20 Minutes

Servings: 8

Ingredients

Roasted Brussels Sprouts:

- 3 cups Brussels sprouts , ends trimmed, yellow leaves removed
- 3 tablespoons olive oil
- Salt to taste
- Roasted Butternut Squash:
- 1 ½ lb butternut squash peeled, seeded, and cubed into 1-inch cubes (Yields about 4 cups of uncooked cubed butternut squash)
- 2 tablespoons olive oil
- 3 tablespoons maple syrup
- ½ teaspoon ground cinnamon

Other Ingredients:

- ½ cups pumpkin seeds

- 1 cup dried cranberries
- 2-4 tablespoons maple syrup optional

Instructions

Roasted Brussels sprouts:

1. Preheat oven to 400 F. Lightly grease the foil-lined baking sheet with 1 tablespoon of olive oil.
2. Make sure Brussels sprouts have trimmed ends and yellow leaves are removed. Then, slice all Brussels sprouts in half. In a medium bowl, combine halved Brussels sprouts, 2 tablespoons of olive oil, salt (to taste), and toss to combine. Place onto a foil-lined baking sheet, cut side down, and roast in the oven at 400 F for about 20-25 minutes. During the last 5-10 minutes of roasting, turn them over for even browning, the cut sides should be nicely and partially charred but not blackened (see my photos).

Roasted butternut squash:

1. Preheat oven to 400 F. Lightly grease the foil-lined baking sheet with 1 tablespoon of olive oil.

2. In a medium bowl, combine cubed butternut squash (peeled and seeded),1 tablespoon of olive oil, maple syrup, and cinnamon, and toss to mix.

3. Place butternut squash in a single layer on the baking sheet. Bake for 20-25 minutes, turning once half-way through baking, until softened.

4. You can roast both Brussels sprouts and butternut squash on 2 separate baking sheets at the same time, on the same rack in the oven – that's what I did.

Assembly:

1. In a large bowl, combine roasted Brussels sprouts, roasted butternut squash, pumpkin seeds, and cranberries, and mix to combine. (OPTIONAL): For more sweetness, add 2 or 4 tablespoons of maple syrup, if desired – do not add all maple syrup at once, start with 2 tablespoons, then add more, if desired, and toss with the salad ingredients to combine.

Prep Time: 20 Minutes

Cook Time: 20 Minutes

Servings: 6

Ingredients

- 1 tablespoon olive oil
- lb chicken breasts , thinly sliced
- 1 onion , chopped
- 4 garlic cloves , minced
- 1 teaspoon cumin
- salt
- 2 cups chicken broth
- 2 tablespoons chili powder
- 4 oz green chili peppers, , chopped, from the can
- 15 oz pinto beans , undrained, from the can
- 15 oz chickpeas (garbanzo beans), from the can
- 15 oz corn , drained, from the can
- 15 oz refried pinto beans , from the can, or 1 extra can (15 oz) of great northern beans, pureed
- 1 cup Cheddar shredded, or Mexican cheese, shredded
- 4 green onions , chopped

Instructions

2. Heat the oil in a large soup pot over medium heat. Add the sliced chicken breasts, chopped onion, minced garlic, ½ teaspoon cumin and salt to taste, and saute on medium heat for about 5 minutes, constantly stirring, until onion is soft and meat is no longer pink.

3. Cut up the cooked chicken into even thinner slices so that it looks like it's shredded.

4. Add chicken broth, green chili peppers, remaining cumin (½ teaspoon), 1 tablespoon chili powder, pinto beans, garbanzo beans, corn, and refried pinto beans.

5. Stir everything well, making sure refried pinto beans are evenly incorporated in the chili, making it thick.

6. If you don't have a can of refried beans, use an extra 1 can (15 oz) of pinto beans (or any white bean), pureed. The idea of adding refried beans or pureed beans is to thicken the chili. Add more chili powder if needed.

7. Bring to boil, make sure to stir all ingredients well together to combine flavors and spices. Reduce to simmer and cook for 15 minutes on simmer, constantly stirring, until the chili thickens.

8. Serve in soup bowls, garnished with shredded Cheddar or Mexican cheese, sour creams, and chopped green onion.

Prep Time: 30 Minutes

Cook Time: 30 Minutes

Servings: 14

Ingredients

Spaghetti squash fritters:

- 2 eggs
- ⅔ cup flour (for gluten free version, use multi-purpose gluten-free King Arthur flour)
- 2 cups spaghetti squash , cooked and wringed out (see below)
- 2 cups quinoa , cooked
- ½ cup Parmesan cheese shredded
- ¼ cup spinach fresh, finely chopped (OPTIONAL)
- ¼ teaspoon salt
- 6 strips bacon , cooked, drained of fat, and chopped
- 2 tablespoons vegetable oil or olive oil

For garnish:

- 2 green onions chopped
- dollop of sour cream or Greek Yogurt

Instructions

How to cook spaghetti squash

1. The recipe requires 2 CUPS COOKED spaghetti squash. First 5 steps describe how to cook spaghetti squash (this can be done 1 or more days in advance):
2. Preheat oven to 425 Fahrenheit.
3. Cut the squash in 2 halves, scrape out the seeds and the fiber out of each half. Spray oil over the cut sides of the squash. Spray the baking sheet with oil and place the squash on the baking sheet cut side down.
4. Bake for about 30-40 minutes. Remove it from the oven when it's cooked through and soft, and let it cool. Flip the squash so that cut side faces up – that will speed up the cooling. After squash cools, scrape squash with a fork to remove flesh in long strands and transfer to a bowl. Let it cool.
5. Important: Wring out the spaghetti squash by wrapping small portions of it in paper towels and squeezing hard with your hands over the sink. Be careful not to drop the spaghetti squash into the sink if the paper towel breaks. Try to get rid of as much liquid as you can.
6. Cooked spaghetti squash can be refrigerated for 5 days. I prefer to cook spaghetti squash, refrigerate it

and make fritters the next day or 2 days later - that allows spaghetti squash to drain the liquid out and get dryer, which is preferable for fritters.

How to make fritters:

1. In a large bowl, using electric mixer, beat 2 eggs on high speed for 1-2 minutes. Add flour and continue beating for about 30 seconds to combine. To the same bowl, add spaghetti squash, quinoa, Parmesan cheese, finely chopped spinach,and ¼ teaspoon of salt. Mix very well until all the mixture has uniform consistency. Add chopped bacon and mix. Taste and adjust seasoning, if necessary.

2. Heat a large skillet on high-medium heat until VERY hot. Only then add oil. It should sizzle and smoke right away.

3. Using a tablespoon, spoon the tablespoon-ful of the batter for each fritter and drop on the skillet. Using a spatula, correct the shape of each fritter, making it flatter and rounder. Cook until the bottom side of each fritter is golden brown, about 1-2 minutes. Reduce heat to medium.

4. Using spatula, flip fritters to the opposite side, and cook 1-2 more minutes. When flipping the fritters, you

can use a spoon on the opposite side of spatula to help push each fritter onto the spatula and then flipping.

5. Turn off the heat and let the fritters sit in the skillet (uncovered) for 2-3 more minutes (check the bottom to make sure it's not burned - if it is too dark, remove fritters from the skillet immediately). Do 4 fritters at a time.

6. Serve as is, or top with the dollop of sour cream or Greek yogurt and chopped green onions (delicious if served this way!).

Prep Time: 20 Minutes

Cook Time: 30 Minutes

Servings: 4

Ingredients

- 1 tablespoon olive oil
- 1 pound ground beef
- 1 onion , chopped
- 4 garlic cloves , minced
- 1 cup pumpkin puree , from the can or homemade
- 1 cup tomatoes , from the can
- 1 cup vegetable stock or water
- 15 oz black beans , from the can, drained
- 1 teaspoon cumin powder
- 1 teaspoon chili powder
- ¼ teaspoon salt , at least

Garnish

- ½ cup cheddar cheese , shredded
- ½ cup mozzarella cheese , shredded
- 4 green onions , chopped

- ¼ cup sour cream , optional

Instructions

1. In a large pot or skillet, heat olive oil, add the ground beef, chopped onion and minced garlic and cook for about 5 minutes on medium heat until onion is soft and meat is no longer pink. Drain.

2. Add pumpkin, canned tomatoes (chop them up into smaller chunks), vegetable stock (or water), black beans (drained). Add 1 teaspoon of cumin, 1 teaspoon of chili powder, and ¼ teaspoon salt, stir everything well, and season with more salt if needed.

3. Bring to boil, make sure to stir all ingredients well together to combine flavors and spices. Reduce to simmer and cook pumpkin beef chili for 15 minutes on simmer.

4. Serve pumpkin chili in soup bowls, garnished with shredded cheeses, chopped green onion, and, optionally, sour cream.

28. Quinoa Salad with Roasted Butternut Squash, Feta, and Pine Nuts

Prep Time: 30 Minutes

Cook Time: 20 Minutes

Servings: 6

Ingredients

- 1 ½ cups quinoa , cooked
- 1 onion , sliced
- ½ butternut squash , medium size
- 3 tablespoons olive oil
- salt
- ¼ cup French Vinaigrette salad dressing , add generous amounts of dressing to individual portions
- ¼ cup Feta cheese
- ¼ cup pine nuts , toasted

Instructions

How to roast butternut squash:

1. Preheat the oven to 400 F. Line the baking sheet with aluminum foil and grease with 1 tablespoon of olive oil.

2. Peel the squash and slice it into ¾ inch cubes. You will only need ½ of the medium size squash. Toss the squash cubes in a large bowl with 2 tablespoons olive oil and generously sprinkle with salt.

3. Put butternut squash on the greased baking sheet and roast for about 30 minutes, until soft. Flip the squash cubes over midway through baking. Let it cool slightly before adding to the salad.

How to caramelize onions:

1. Caramelize onions according to the instructions here.

Assembling quinoa salad:

2. In a large bowl, combine cooked quinoa, roasted butternut squash, caramelized onions, and mix with the dressing. Add the dressing only before the serving, and add as much as you want to individual portions, as both quinoa and butternut squash tend to be on a dry side, and this dressing (when generously applied) fixes this beautifully!

3. Top each individual serving of quinoa salad with Feta cheese and toasted pine nuts.

4. The quinoa salad keeps very well refrigerated for up to a week, but only without dressing. Add the dressing only before serving.

Prep Time: 20 Minutes

Cook Time: 30 Minutes

Servings: 6

Ingredients

Quinoa Chili:

- 1 cup quinoa , uncooked
- 1 tablespoon olive oil
- 1 onion , chopped
- 4 garlic cloves , minced
- 2 cups tomatoes , from the can
- 2 cups pumpkin puree ,from the can or homemade
- 2 cups water
- 15 oz black beans , from the can, drained
- 15 oz garbanzo beans , from the can, drained
- 1 tablespoon cumin
- 2 tablespoons chili powder
- ½ salt at least

Garnish:

- sour cream

- ½ cup cheddar cheese , shredded
- ½ cup mozzarella cheese , shredded
- 4 green onions , chopped

Instructions

Quinoa:

1. Add 1 cup of quinoa and 2 cups of water to a large pan.
2. Bring to boil. Reduce heat.
3. Simmer for about 15 minutes until the quinoa absorbs the water.

Quinoa Chili

1. In a large pot or skillet, cook the chopped onion and minced garlic in olive oil for about 2 minutes on medium heat until the onion is soft.
2. Add pumpkin, canned tomaStoes (chop them up into smaller chunks), water, black beans (drained), garbanzo beans (drained), quinoa.
3. Add 1 tablespoon of cumin, 2 tablespoons of chili powder, and ½ and ¼ teaspoon salt.
4. Stir everything well, and season with more salt if needed.

5. Bring to boil.

6. Stir all the ingredients well together to combine flavors and spices. Reduce to simmer and cook pumpkin quinoa chili for 15 minutes on simmer.

7. Serve in soup bowls, garnished with sour cream, shredded cheeses, and chopped green onion.

Prep Time: 15 Minutes

Cook Time: 30 Minutes

Servings: 6

Ingredients

- 1 lb pork sausage
- 2 bell peppers , diced
- 8 oz elbow macaroni , dry
- 18 oz marinara sauce
- 18 oz water
- ⅓ cup half and half
- ⅓ cup mozzarella cheese

Instructions

1. In a large skillet cook sausage on medium heat, until meat is brown. Drain off fat.
2. Add diced bell peppers, dried elbow macaroni, marinara sauce, and water. Bring to boil; reduce heat to simmer. Simmer, covered, for about 20 minutes until macaroni is tender, occasionally stirring.

3. Add half and half, sprinkle with cheese, and mix everything well. Remove from heat, cover and let it sit for about 2 minutes or until cheese melts.